The Dynamite Story of Alzheimer's Recoveries

By Allen K. Golden, BA Ed

A Practical Guide to Alzheimer's Disease

A medical fairytale comes true! Read about 27 factual doctor research studies on Alzheimer's Disease.

Read the story of the six U.S. Patents and one international patent.

Read the story of the doctor whose husband had a 3 year battle with dementia. When she put him in a clinical trial and found and converted medication to a holistic treatment, 16 months later her husband was able to work in a medical warehouse. In August of 2010 I talked to this doctor and she stated that this is the sixth year of his illness and it is wonderful. He only cannot drive due to challenges of quick responses common with Alzheimer's Disease.

All material in this book is provided for information only and should not be construed as medical advice or instruction. No action should be taken solely on the contents of this book. Patients and caregivers should consult their appropriate health care physicians on any matter relating to their own health and well-being.

The Dynamite Story of Alzheimer's Recoveries

By Allen K. Golden, BA Ed

A Practical Guide to Alzheimer's Disease

Revised April 20, 2011

ISBN 978-0-615-48015-2
Contact Information:

Allen K. Golden
Seek Health Ltd.
2008 West Broadway
Suite 152
Council Bluffs, IA 51501

allenkgolden@yahoo.com

All material in this book is provided for information only and should not be construed as medical advice or instruction. No action should be taken solely on the contents of this book. Patients and caregivers should consult their appropriate health care physicians on any matter relating to their own health and well-being.

Table of Contents

Appendix

I feel blessed by being the person who can deliver this huge message of recovery to the Alzheimer's patients who desperately need the help that this book provides.

Additionally, I would like to thank three of my friends who helped me compile the material, edits, and typing involved to finish this work. Namely, Jenny Blevins, Cheryl Kent, and Lisa Tomey are so gratefully thanked for their efforts in completing this book.

This book is not intended to provide medical advice, diagnosis or treatment. Consultation with a qualified medical professional is recommended.

The Journey

I have had serious health problems since 1960. I have suffered from chronic fatigue from the pesticide Chloradane and internal poisoning from massive doses of penicillin, taken for an infection in my leg. The friendly flora in my body was killed. Within a week I was reduced to about 10 percent of normal energy.

Since that time, I have spent approximately half a million dollars, out-of-pocket, in order to find ways to keep myself functioning. I have been all over the United States, Canada and Mexico trying to find help for my condition. Over the past ten years I have subscribed to about eight alternative, physician monthly newsletters. As a result, I have learned many of their new findings and places to treat many of the unusual maladies that can happen to people.

In order to find help for myself, I do a lot of research. I want to share my findings and hope to contribute to the wellness and health of other affected individuals. This research has provided some astounding material about Alzheimer's Disease. Also mentioned are diagnoses such as Parkinson's, Multiple Sclerosis, Autism, and Amyotrophic Lateral Sclerosis (ALS) (Also known as Lou Gehrig's Disease). These are closely related to similar symptoms and could be helped by the same method of therapy. I was surprised to find that much of the research started back before the year 2000.

As modern science goes, it is normally 10 to 20 years before anyone has knowledge of the material. After this, it can take another 10 years or longer before the information becomes available to the consumer.

The articles I have researched have made me aware that only a handful of scientists and a few others in the drug industry knew of these tremendous findings. After I received three of these new reports on Alzheimer's Disease, I went to the medical libraries in Omaha, Nebraska. I continued to research and organize findings about neurological disorders.

One thing that ties many of the neurological disorders together is that the neurons are damaged. This is due in part to nutrition and pathogens which prevent normal functioning of the brain. These diseases have been termed "diabetes of the brain." The amazing fact is that the brain neurons are damaged and the use of coconut oil is causing recovery. This book is my effort to put information in an easy to understand approach. It is with empathy for those who are facing Alzheimer's Disease, whether as a patient or caregiver, to have information at hand which can be quickly applied.

A close friend who I discussed this book with shared her story about her experience with Alzheimer's. Her father was diagnosed with Alzheimer's in 2003. He was 83 at the time. He was put on Aricept and Namenda along with his medications for diabetes and high blood pressure. What my friend noticed earlier in life is that her father had signs of memory confusion in the home in his late 40's. It was small things such as remembering names. He still had the mental clarity to perform complex functions in his job. As the years went on there started to be problems with work performance. Eventually he had to take an early retirement. When he started exhibiting dangerous behaviors such as speeding while driving and acting like it was funny concerns started up.

Eventually he had an accident which he never recalled. His license was eventually revoked with the assistance of family members. This was after a complete neurological exam diagnosed him with Alzheimer's. He was in denial about this disease and eventually ended up in assisted living due to being in a non structured, unsupervised situation. Once the medications were given and monitored more closely he showed some degree of improvement. My friend wishes that the news about treatments was known at that time. Perhaps his life would have been enriched, even at the stage he entered. She is very enthused about these studies regarding Alzheimer's Disease.

Alzheimer's Disease

What is Alzheimer's Disease?

The Centers for Disease Control and Prevention (CDC) offers this definition:

> "Alzheimer's disease is the most common form of dementia among older adults. Alzheimer's disease involves parts of the brain that control thought, memory, and language and can seriously affect a person's ability to carry out daily activities. Although scientists are learning more every day, right now, they still do not know what causes Alzheimer's disease." (1)

Who Gets Alzheimer's Disease?

Upwards of five million people have been diagnosed with Alzheimer's Disease in the United States alone. Expected to have on onset at about age 60, it still can show up sooner. As people age past 60 the chance of being diagnosed increases. Once the age of 85 is reached the chances are 50:50 that Alzheimer's Disease will be diagnosed. (1) It is important to note that this does not mean that Alzheimer's Disease is inevitable.

Risk Factors for Alzheimer's Disease

Age is the most common risk factor associated with Alzheimer's Disease but genetics go hand in hand with this factor. It is possible to get Alzheimer's Disease before retirement age but this is only true for a small percentage of cases. (2)

Cardiovascular Disease fed by high cholesterol and/or high blood pressure have been found to contribute to damages resulting in dementia. Type 2 Diabetes also comes in as a contender for an introduction to Alzheimer's Disease. (2) Insulin resistance affects the brain and is one of the reasons Alzheimer's Disease is sometimes called Type 3 Diabetes.

Diet and exercise have come forth as linking to better health over all. Eating whole grains, fruits, vegetables, less sugar and less food additives have been found to help with prevention of illnesses which contribute to Alzheimer's Disease. (2)

Normal adults must have proper metabolism of glucose for brain energy. Amino acids are essential to be supplied by diet alone. This comes with one exception. The brain can also use metabolism of ketone bodies for energy. (3)

Recent research sponsored by the National Institute on Aging and the National Institute of Neurological Disorders and Stroke has brought forward awareness of the hereditary factor of Alzheimer's. Robyn Honea of the University of Kansas School of Medicine led the study. Findings were that of the test group there was a significant amount of gray matter in patients who had a mother who had Alzheimer's. This was as much as double that of the participants who had a father or no relative with Alzheimer's. The participants were all free of dementia. The conclusion was that when a mother has Alzheimer's the likelihood to develop the disease is 4 to 10 times greater. (17)

The foods you eat contribute to Alzheimer's. It is sometimes called diabetes of the brain. Having diabetes or pre-diabetes can be a pre-cursor to getting Alzheimer's. Suzanne de la Monte , M.D., M.P.H. Associate Professor of Pathology and Medicine, states that diabetes can form in various organs in the body, including the brain. Insulin then becomes an important concern. Genetic factors are only one indicator of potential Alzheimer's. There is also an alarming increase in diagnoses of Alzheimer's which overrides genetics. (21)

The four food groups which can affect Alzheimer's due to nitrosoamines AKA sodium nitrite are smoked meats, processed cheese, some beers which contain nitrosomines, white rice, and white flour. Nitrosoamines are preservatives which may be in these processed foods. (22)

Prevention and Treatment for Alzheimer's Disease

Do proper diet or dietary supplements prevent and cure Alzheimer's Disease? More studies have been completed and others in process which answer this question. Case studies such as that of Mary Newport, M.D. conducted with her husband, Steve who Dr. Newport has been treating his Alzheimer's with coconut oil, medium chain triglycerides (MCT), omega 3 fish oil capsules, and two meals of salmon a week. This has brought about a remarkable change. (4)

MCT oil is a product which is reformulated from coconut oil in order to remove the grease. This is preferred by many people. However, it is important to keep in mind that coconut oil in the virgin form is best for accessing all essential amino acids for treatment.

Despite the genetic and physical diversity in the causes of Alzheimer's and Parkinson's Diseases, findings indicate that ketones can protect neurons in the forms of these diseases and indicate that the two conditions have common features. (5) The features are body dementia, impairment of energy metabolism,(6) hypoperfusion (the transfer of fluid through a tissue) (7) or trauma. (8)

Fat is the main energy source of a newborn baby. It provides 50 percent of the total calories in human milk and formula. Fats are imperative to normal development because they provide the fatty acids needed for brain development. These energy lipids can be stored by the body to no limits in contrast to limited storage capacity for carbohydrates and proteins. (10)

Before birth, glucose is the main source of energy for the fetus, whereas the fetal requirements for fatty acids are mainly supplied as free fatty acids from the mother. After birth, fat is supplied chiefly in the form of milk triglycerides.

Data seems to indicate that mother's milk is highly valuable to the newborn. Mother's milk passes on immunities and triglycerides (a lipid or neutral fat comprising glycerol and three fatty-acid molecules). (11)

Triglycerides are one of the components which fuel the body. Triglycerides are manufactured in the body from the digested products of fat in the diet. Fats are stored in the body as triglycerides which contain 98 to 99 percent of the total milk fat in the form of membrane-enclosed milk fat globules. The globule membrane is composed mostly of phospholipids, cholesterol, and proteins. However, the core of a globule is composed mainly of triglycerides. Like the glucose function is to help energize the body, the triglycerides do similar roles in giving the body energy when glucose is not doing its proper job. (12)

Glucose is the main source of energy for the human body generated by a low carbohydrate diet with a low glycemic index. Glucose alone is not able to maintain the body's energy source. Triglycerides are needed to help the brain function at a better level.

The early nutrients of milk appear to have been lost as the person ages. The body may get more toxic due to eating habits, food selection and lifestyle. This all can add to the problems associated with Alzheimer's and other neuro-related brain diseases. It all seems to go back to where we arrive at the basic energy source.

Richard L. Veech, M.D. and George F. Cahill, Jr. M.D. have completed extensive studies regarding therapeutic effects in relation to ketosis. As success has been shown with the ketogenic diet, it is a difficult diet to maintain for any great length of time. It is hopeful that there will be funding available to allow manufacture of the pharmaceutic treatment proposed by Doctors Veech and Cahill. (16) More about this research will be discussed in further reading.

Research by the Monell Center found that "Oleocanthal, a naturally-occurring compound found in extra-virgin olive oil, alters the structure of neurotoxic proteins believed to contribute to the debilitating effects of Alzheimer's disease. This structural change impedes the proteins' ability to damage brain nerve cells. Future studies to identify more precisely how oleocanthal changes ADDL structure may increase understanding of the pharmacological actions of oleocanthal, ibuprofen, and structurally related plant compounds. Such pharmacological insights could provide discovery pathways related to disease prevention and treatment." (18)

Another study found that Resveratrol, a compound found in grapes, red wine, peanuts and berries, lowers the levels of the amyloid-beta peptides, which cause much of the neurological damage associated with Alzheimer's disease. More is to be found on this topic but this offers hope for Alzheimer's and other human amyloid related diseases, including Huntington's and Parkinson's. (19)

Dr. Frank Shallenberger Delves into the Unknown

Frank Shallenberger, M.D., H.M.D. from Norcross, Georgia is in the forefront for finding help for his Alzheimer's patients. He found that the most effective way of increasing the body's production of more ketones was by introducing a diet low in carbohydrates. In an article in the Journal Neurotherapeutics Dr. Shallenberger shared about how they went about proving their theory. (15)

Researchers administered the Alzheimer's Disease Assessment Scale (ADAS). This test measures the memory performance, along with other aspects of brain performance. The study had very impressive results. When the blood ketone levels of Alzheimer's patients was increased for only three months, the ADAS-Cog scores did not decline. They actually increased. Compared to patients in the control group whose ketone levels remained unchanged during the same time period, their scores declined significantly. What's more, when the researchers allowed the ketone levels of the treated patients to decrease back to normal, their scores dropped accordingly. (15)

The use of virgin, organic, pharmaceutic level coconut oil will increase ketones. Fatty acids are absorbed quickly in the intestines, then on to the liver and on to result in ketones. Dr. Shallenberger relates to the story of Steve Newport and how his wife, Dr. Mary Newport, started her husband on the coconut oil and documented the progress. An actual test of the theory proved positive results. (15)

As we age, the brain's ability to convert glucose into energy decreases. When the brain uses energy from ketones the brain's ability to energize is not impaired. Actually, the results are a marked improvement. The regimen Dr. Shallenberger has suggested is to use 2 tablespoons of virgin coconut oil twice a day. This can be mixed with hot water, blended in smoothies, mixed with oatmeal and more. (15)

When the diet is supplemented with MCT and coconut oil the conversion to ketones occurs without any other dietary change. In other words you can have your carbs and ketones too! This direct conversion of fatty acids to ketones is why coconut oil is so healthy. It is also what makes coconut oil such a fantastic treatment for Alzheimer's.

Dr. Julian Whitaker – The Giant Breakthrough

Julian Whitaker, M.D. developed the Whitaker Wellness Institute for the purpose of helping people who have not had success with conventional medical treatments. He recommends a daily walking regimen to help with disease prevention. Proper nutrition which includes highly nutritious vegetables, fruit, legumes, and whole grains. Dr. Whitake has found that low dose Naltrexone has benefits for Alzheimer's as well as autoimmune disorders.

Dr. Whitaker also recommends adding omega-3-rich fish often and poultry and lean protein for other meals. As an attack against free radicals the following dosages are suggested: 1,500 mg vitamin C, 400-800 IU vitamin E, 5,000 IU vitamin A, and 15,000 IU beta-carotene. As a way to help methylation Dr. Whitaker recommends: 800 mcg folic acid, 150 mcg vitamin B12, and 75 mg vitamin B6. Taking two fish oil capsules per day can also help inflammation. (20) Weight loss is imperative if there is any obesity.

Dr. Jonathan Wright – Phenomenal Findings About Nutrition

Jonathan V. Wright, M.D. says that lithium is the mineral no brain should be without. Lithium is a natural occurring mineral. Lithium is potentially protective against Alzheimer's disease. Alzheimer's patients also suffer neural cell loss and increased cortical levels. Lithium was found to inhibit an enzyme called "GSK-3" (glycogen synthase kinase 3) which acts to add phosphate molecules. This process is called phosphorylation to a nerve cell structure called tau protein. Phosphorylation is a very common biochemical in our bodies, but in Alzheimer's disease tau protein is hyperactive. Many Alzheimer's patients with dementia have prominent cortical changes with abundant neural-fibrillary tangles with neuritic plaques.

Lithium prevents the formation of these neuralfibrillary tangles which helps to prevent Alzheimer's. (14)

Dr. Wright discusses the use of about 10 to 20 milligrams of Lithium for Alzheimer's prevention. He also suggests using about one tablespoon of fish oil daily. This works as an anti-inflammatory and will help put a hold on cancer and heart disease. Omega-3 fatty acids also provide repair of brain cell membranes. The use of hormones as a suggested prevention is more individualized and requires medical monitoring by a doctor who specializes in nutrition. He recommends checking on acam.org or calling American College for Advancement in Medicine at (800) 532-3688 to find physicians who specialize in these treatments. (13)

Another mineral very important to Alzheimer's prevention is niacinamide. Researchers from the University of California, Irvine, discovered that niacinamide successfully treated and in fact - REVERSED – early Alzheimer's disease in experimental animals. They noted a 60 percent reduction in the tau protein in the animals brain cells. In the next few years, niacinamide will be found very important in Alzheimer's disease prevention. (14)

There are major components in some foods which can reduce the risk of Alzheimer's. The yellow spice turmeric has a compound called curcumin, which has specific actions that can reduce the risk of Alzheimer's disease. Ginger and cayenne are also good for fighting inflammation in the body.(14)

There have been more studies about new options as well as some treatments which help delay Alzheimer's. While there are more efforts made to lock down a cure, there are also approaches which can be attempted in the meantime. We will learn more about combinations of medications and other treatment approaches which seem to work best for Alzheimer's patients.

There are currently five FDA approved medications for Alzheimer's. They are: Donepezil or Aricept ® which is used at all stages of Alzheimer's, Galantamine or Razadyne ® for mild to moderate levels of the disease, Memantine or Namenda ® for moderate to severe levels, Rivastigmine or Exelon ® for mild to moderate levels, and Tacrine or Cognex ® for mild to moderate levels. The five Alzheimer's medications help for about 6 to 12 months for about 50 percent of patients.

Medications which are used for slowing down Alzheimer's are Donepezil, Galantamine, Rivastigmine and Tacrine. These are called Cholinedterase inhibitors. Memantine is a NMDA Receptor Antagonist. This drug regulates glutamate. Too much glutamate causes a calcium blockage to the cell surfaces. Memantine partially blocks the NMDA receptors. (12)

As caregivers and Alzheimer's disease patients search for solutions for this challenging disease there is hope. There are new developments through research and drug trials. To check on drug trial information you can go to alz.org and click on "find a clinical trial." You can then search for clinical trials which may be a match. You can also call (800) 272-3900 for the same service. (12) More clinical trials for Alzheimer's Disease can be located by going to clinicaltrials.gov

Points to Review

➢ A thorough physical workup is in order. This would include checking for cholesterol levels, diabetes, kidney and liver functions. Ask about lithium levels to determine if lithium treatment is necessary.

➢ Consider consultation with a wholeness nutritionist regarding supplements and nutrition. If weight loss is in order, request guidance. Ask about resveratrol as a supplement.

➢ Eat whole grains and complex carbohydrates such as found in whole fruits and vegetables. Avoid sugars and additives as much as possible. Add about 2-3 meals of wild salmon per week. You can also use snapper, cod, and shrimp. Avoid tuna, halibut and non-wild salmon due to a greater risk for metal toxicity.

➢ Only cook with saturated fats. These are fats which are generally solid at room temperature. Coconut oil is a good first choice but it does tend to smoke at above 325. The preferred method of cooking fish is to bake or broil since frying will remove the benefits of omega3. Squash, walnuts, flax-seed, navy and kidney beans also provide substantial omega3.

➢ Take 2 fish oil capsules per day with a meal for inflammation. Consider using turmeric, cayenne, or ginger when cooking.

➢ Exercise the body and the mind on a daily basis. Do things differently such as using the opposing hands to complete a task. Try games and activities which challenge the brain. Involving family and friends makes this fun.

➢ Diabetics should monitor blood glucose levels regularly. Adjust diet and medications according to guidance of a physician.

➢ Approach soy products cautiously as the majority are genetically modified and may not respond well with your system. There are many other good types of protein to consider.

➢ Soy blocks the use of fat soluble vitamins. (See "Soy Alert" of the Weston Price Foundation).

➢ Add virgin coconut oil to the diet. This comes in various sizes and the usual first start is in 8 ounce containers. It looks like a solid shortening. Use in place of butter and other fats in the diet. Treatment levels are about 2 tablespoons at least twice per day. This may vary and more is not normally considered harmful. Keep in mind that this always needs to be made available in the body to work continuously. Eating with roughage such as salad with help keep the coconut oil working in the intestines longer.

➢ Consider checking for resources at the American College for Advancement in Medicine at (800) 532-3688 or alz.org Also you can go to clinicaltrials.gov

➢ Call (800) 272-3900 to check on clinical trials.

References:

1. **Centers for Disease Control and Prevention, 1600 Clifton Rd., Atlanta, GA 30333** www.cdc.gov

2. **American Health Assistance Foundation, 22512 Gateway Center Drive, Clarksburg, MD 20871** www.ahaf.org

3. **Newport, Mary M.D., *What if there was a cure for Alzheimer's Disease and no one knew?* 2008**

4. **Dunnet, Stephen B. and others, Cell therapy in Parkinson's disease – stop or go? *Nature Reviews-Neuroscience,* 365-369**

5. **Gabuzda, Dana and Other, Inhibition of Energy Metabolism Alters the Processing off Amyloid Precursor Protein and Induces a Potentially Amyloidogenicc Derivative, *The Journal of Biological Chemistry,* 1994. 13623-13628**

6. **Kalaria, R.N. and Others, The New York Academy of Sciences 695, 190-193**

7. **Graham, D.I,. and Others, Acta Neurochirurgica, Wein, Supp. 66, 96-102**

8. **Gerngross, T.U. National Biotechnology, 1999, 17, 541-542**

9. **Hamosh, M. and Hamosh, P., Lipoprotein lipase: Its physiological and clinical significance. *Mol Aspects Med* 1983, 6, 199-289**

10. **Hamosh, Margit PhD and Others, Lipids in milk and first steps in their digestion, *Feeding the Normal Infant,* 2001**

11. **Patton, S. Keenan, T.W., The milk fat globule membrane, *Biochem Biophys Acta,* 1975, 415, 273-309**

12. **Alzheimer's Association, 225 N. Michigan Ave., Fl. 17, Chicago, IL 60601-7633** www.alz.org

13. **Wright, Jonathan, A three-pronged attack on Alzheimer's, *Nutrition and Healing Newletters,* September 23, 2009**

14. **Wright, Jonathan, *Nutrition & Healing Newsletters,* Vol. 16, Issue 8, October 2009**

15. Shallenberger, Frank M.D., Real Cures Newsletter, December 2009

16. Cahill, George F. Jr., M.D. and Veech, Richard L. M.D., Ketoacids? Good Medicine?, Transactions of the American Clinical and Climatological Association, Vol 114, 2003

17. Honea, Robyn and others, Progressive regional atrophy in normal adults with a maternal history of Alzheimer disease, *Neurology*, Vol. 76 no. 9 822-829, March 1, 2011

18. Monell Chemical Senses Center. "Natural Compound In Extra-virgin OliveOil -- Oleocanthal -- May Help Prevent, Treat Alzheimer's." ScienceDaily September 29, 2009

19. Marambaud, Philippe and Others, Resveratrol Promotes Clearance of Alzheimer's Disease AmyloidB-Peptides, *J. Biol. Chem.* Vol. 280; Issue 45: 37377-37382

20. Whitaker, Julian M.D. www.whitakerwellness.com

21. de la Monte, SM and Wands, JR, Alzheimer's disease is type 3 diabetes-evidence reviewed. *J Diabetes Sci Technol.* 2008 Nov;2(6):1101-13.

22. Oz, Mehmet www.doctoroz.com

Research and Patent information for Treatment of Alzheimer's Disease and Other Reduced Neuronal Metabolism Diseases by Samuel Henderson and Team

Phenomenal research has been conducted by Samuel Henderson and his team, as supported by Accera, Inc. This patent application by Accera, Inc. and Samuel Henderson, Inventor, is found under Application Number PCT/US2007/072499. The filing date was June 27, 2007 and updated in 2010. This is an international patent application which includes several countries and states.

The title of this patent is: "Combinations of Medium Chain Triglycerides and Therapeutic Agents for the Treatment and Prevention of Alzheimer's Disease and Other Diseases Resulting from Reduced Neuronal Metabolism."

The abstract of the patent introduces that the use of therapeutic agents could improve cognitive abilities. The use of donepezil, rivastigmine, galatamine, and memantive can be used as such therapeutic agents. These agents work against Alzheimer's, obesity, diabetes, hypertension, inflammation and any combinations of these diseases or illnesses. The key is the correct administration of triglycerides and fatty acids.

More specifically this invention offers a treatment for: "Alzheimer's Disease, Mild Cognitive Impairment, and other diseases associated with reduced neuronal metabolism, including Parkinson's Disease, Huntington's Disease, and Epilepsy."

There are no current therapeutic agents to effectively treat or prevent Alzheimer's. There are several medications which mainly utilize functional nerve cells to offer some symptomatic relief. These medications are: Aricept ®, Cognex ®. Reminyl ®/Razadine ®, Exelon ®, and Namenda ®.

Decreased neuronal metabolism has been found to be a culprit for Alzheimer's Disease besides the Cholinergic systems which are considered the main factors of the disease. Glucose metabolism, which could be detected before Alzheimer's Disease, is a large factor of treating this disease. Once Alzheimer's is diagnosed, it has been found that working with the ineffective metabolism of glucose can result in Alzheimer's improvement. It has been evaluated that the insulin resistance to the brain may be a big factor of Alzheimer's, such as it is with diabetes. The liver is not aware of what is happening in the brain and will not process fatty acids. Without the ketone bodies the neurons in the brain of an Alzheimer's patient may starve to death.

Attempts to use insulin as part of the treatment of Alzheimer's patients have been known to produce challenging complications. This led to the need for an agent which could provide better metabolic treatment for Alzheimer's. Under normal condition the brain relies on glucose for energy. Glucose is not something which can be stored in the brain. Neurons do not store glucose. Without the flow of glucose to the brain the result is damaged neurons. If gradual reduction in glucose occurs, the brain will metabolize ketone bodies. This replaces the glucose so that no neuron damage can occur.

High carbohydrate diets tend to reduce the manufacture of ketone bodies. The liver basically stops metabolism of fats. Obesity and other health issues occur from these kinds of diets. Insulin levels increase and stay high and fatty acids are not effectively used for energy. This results with fat being stored. Ketone levels stay low. When fasting, following a diabetic plan, or a low carbohydrate diet, ketone levels rise to the demand for energy and are utilized. Fat stores are reduced and the brain gets needed fuel.

Due to the complications due to poor glucose utilization in the brain, resulting in non production of ketone bodies, the brain starves. The key then becomes finding an agent which can address these impairments.

Enter Medium Chain Triglycerides (MCT) which process is such a way that they can effectively result in ketone production. Patients have shown improvement with MCT.

The use of KETASYN, invented by Samuel T. Henderson and team, has been found to be an effective answer to Alzheimer's Disease. Coordination with other medications for Alzheimer's, diabetes medications, lipid utilization agents, anti-atherosclerotic agents, anti-hypertensive agents, anti-inflammatory agent, anti-obesity agent and combinations produce the desired effects for Alzheimer's patients.

Dietary changes are difficult for Alzheimer's patients, especially due to the tendency to favor carbohydrates. This invention is designed to work without dietary changes. Administration of the medication can be accomplished with anything from pills and suppositories to beverages and foods.

There are several patents which are referred to in the research of this product. They are as follows:

United States Patent Numbers

2,408,345 Refers to anti-obesity agents.
2,503,059 and 2,599,000 Refer to anti-hypertensive agents.

3,381,009; 3,511,836; 3,527,761 Refer to anti-hypertensive agents.
3,752,814 and 3,752,888 Refer to anti-obesity agents.
3,997,666; 4,026,894; 4,046,889 Refer to anti-hypertensive agents.

4,062,950 and 4,174,439 Refer to glucosidase inhibitors.
4,188,390 Refers to anti-hypertensive agents.
4,231,938 "Certain compounds isolated after cultivation of a microorganism belonging to the genus *Aspergillus*, such as lovastatin."
4,248,883 and 4,252,721 Refer to anti-hypertensive agents.
4,254,256 Refers to glucosidase inhibitors.
4,273,765 Refers to amylase inhibitors.
4,315,007; 4,337,201; 4,344,949 Refer to anti-hypertensive agents.
4,346,227 "Discloses ML-236B derivatives, such as pravastatin."
4,374,829 and 4,410,520 Refer to anti-hypertensive agents.

4,444,784 "Discloses synthetic derivatives of compounds isolated after cultivation of a microorganism belonging to the genus *Aspergillus,* such as simvastatin."
4,451,455 Refers to amylase inhibitors.
4,452,790; 4,470,972; 4,508,727; 4,508,729 Refer to anti-hypertensive agents.
4,528,196 Refers to chelating agents for the treatment of iron overload.
4,528,197 "Controlled triglyceride nutrition for hyper catabolic mammals"
4,555,502 and 4,587,258 Refer to anti-hypertensive agents.
4,623,714 Refers to amylase inhibitors.
4,634,765 Refers to glucosidase inhibitors.
4,639,436 Refers to glucosidase inhibitors and anti-hypertensive agents.
4,699,905; 4,701,559 Refer to glucosidase inhibitors.
4,703,063 Refers to anti-hypertensive agents.
4,739,073 "Discloses certain substituted indoles, such as fluvastatin."
4,766,121 and 4,826,876 Refer to thyromimetic agents.
4,847,271 "Discloses certain oxetane compounds."
4,847,296 "Triglyceride preparations for the prevention of catabolism."
4,910,305 Refers to thyromimetic agents.

4,929,629 Refers to anti-obesity agents.

4,933,361 Refers to anti-hypertensive agents.

5,011,859 "Discloses certain fluoro analogs of squalene."

5,026,554 "Discloses fermentation products of the microorganism MF5465 (ATCC 74011) including zaragozic acid."

5,041,432 "Discloses certain 15-substituted lanosterol derivatives."

5,051,531 Refers to anti-oxidant peroxides.

5,051,534 "Discloses certain cyclopropyloxy-squalene derivatives."

5,061,798 Refers to thyromimetic agents.

5,064,856 "Discloses certain spiro-lactone derivatives prepared by cultivating a microorganism (MF5253)."

5,064,864 "Discloses certain fluoro analogs of squalene."

5,084,461 "Discloses certain azadecalin derivatives."

5,091,524 Refers to glucosidase inhibitors.

5,102,915 "Discloses certain cyclopropyloxy-squalene derivatives."

5,120,729 "Discloses certain beta-lactam derivatives."

5,157,116 and 5,192,772 Refer to glucosidase inhibitors.

5,273,995 Regarding atorvastatin and the hemicalcium salt thereof (Lipitor ®).

5,278,171 Refers to inhibitors of cholesterol biosynthesis.

5,284,971 and 5,401,772 Refer to thyromimetic agents.

5,504,078 Refers to glucosidase inhibitors.

5,510,379 "Discloses certain carboxysulfonates."

5,512,548 "Discloses certain polypeptide derivatives having activity as CETP inhibitors."

5,552,412 Refers to raloxifene, lasofoxifene, and other compounds related to lipid level mediation.

5,654,468 and 5,569,674 Refer to thyromimetic agents.

5,728,704 and 5,866,578 "Discloses compounds and a method for treating or preventing diabetic complications by inhibiting the enzyme sorbitol dehydrogenase."

6,037,346 Refers to anti-hypertensive agents.

6,140,343 "Discloses certain polypeptide derivatives having activity as CETP inhibitors."

Ep-A-0463756; EP-A-0526004; EP-A-0595750; EP-A-0995751; EP-A-1092719 Refers to suitable phosphodiesterase inhibitors.

EP Publication 395,768A "Discloses certain substituted allylamine derivatives."

EP-491,226A "Discloses certain pyridyldihydroxyheptenoic acids, such as rivastatin."

14

<u>Belgian Patent</u> No. 893,553 Refers to anti-hypertensive agent moveltopril.

<u>French Patent Publication</u> 2697250 "Discloses squalene cyclase inhibitors."

<u>International Patent Application No.</u>

WO 94/00453 Refers to suitable phosphodiesterase inhibitors.
WO 94/00480 Cholesterol absorption inhibitors.
WO 94/01404 "Discloses certain acyl-piperidines."
WO 99/02159 and WO 00/02550 Refer to anti-obesity agents.
WO 98/03492 Refers to 5-lipoxygenase inhibitors.
WO 98/03493; WO 98/03494; WO 01/05401 Refer to anti-obesity agents.
WO 94/05661; WO 93/0610; WO 93/07124; WO 93/07149 Refer to suitable phosphodiesterase inhibitors.
WO 99/07703 Refers to anti-obesity agents.

WO 94/10150 "Disclose squalene cyclase inhibitors."
WO 96/10559 Refers to urea derivatives having ACAT inhibitory activity.
WO 93/12069-A "Discloses certain amino alcohol derivatives."
WO 00/12075 Refers to anti-hypertensive agents.
WO 93/12095 Refers to suitable phosphodiesterase inhibitors.
WO 01/13112; WO 96/14307; WO 01/14879 Refer to anti-obesity agents.
WO 00/15216 Refers to preparation and use of certain metabolic precursors.
WO 93/16189 Refers to anti-obesity agents.
WO 94/19978 Refers to suitable phosphodiesterase inhibitors.

WO 96/21656 Refers to raloxifene, lasofoxifene, and other compounds related to lipid level mediation.
WO 98/23593 Refers to compounds which inhibit the secretions of triglycerides, cholesteryl ester, and phospholipids.
WO 99/24433 and WO 00/24745 Refer to suitable phosphodiesterase inhibitors.
WO 96/26948 "Disclose urea derivatives having ACAT inhibitory activity."
WO 01/27112 and WO 01/27113 Refer to suitable phosphodiesterase inhibitors.
WO 00/28993 Refers to anti-obesity agents.

WO 99/30697 Refers to phosphodiesterase inhibitors.
WO 96/35671 Refers to anti-obesity agents.
WO 96/39384 and WO 96/39385 Refer to glycogen phosphorylase inhibitors.

WO 96/40640 Refers to compounds which inhibit the secretions of triglycerides, cholesteryl ester, and phospholipids.
WO 96/40660 Refers to neuropeptide Y antagonists.
WO 98/41201 Refers to preparation and use of certain metabolic precursors.
WO 98/49166 and WO 99/54333 Refer to suitable phosphodiesterase inhibitors.
WO 99/54358; WO 99/55679; WO 00/58361 Refer to anti-obesity agents.
WO 00/59510 Refers to methylene dipiperidine derivatives.
WO 99/64002; WO 99/64008; WO 00/74679 Refer to anti-obesity agents.

U.S. Patent Application Serial Number 09/391,152 "Discloses certain polypeptide derivatives having activity as CETP inhibitors."

U.S. Patent Provisional Ser. No. 60/323,995 "Drug Targets for Alzheimer's Disease and Other Diseases Associated with Decreased Neuronal Metabolism." filed September 21, 2001. The Applicant supports that dietary change is not required.

U.S. Patent Publication 2006/0089380 Plaque removal agents, plaque inhibitors, inhibitors of amyloid processing enzymes, et al.

Note:

The bulk of this patent is about 94 pages in length. This has been a summary from a layperson's point of view.

References:

1. Accera, Inc., Henderson, Samuel T. and additional agents of the International Patent Number PT/US07/72499 "Combinations of Medium Chain Triglycerides and Therapeutic Agents for the Treatment and Prevention of Alzheimer's Disease and Other Diseases Resulting from Reduced Neuronal Metabolism" and references as included in this patent.

Ketones or KeyTones?

As the keys to dietary treatment Alzheimer's Disease are ketones it is easy to remember this with the play of words in the title. Let's take a look at this most valuable information which explains the benefits of ketones.

A subject of sub-cortical dementia is a pattern of mental impairment which happens in disorders in which many changes involve sun-cortical structures. Sub-cortical dementia is characterized by forgetfulness. Slowing of thought processes, depression and an inability to manipulate acquired knowledge. Similar symptoms are seen in patients with Alzheimer's Disease and Parkinson's Disease with dementia. (1) These diagnoses certainly show that the brain is starving for energy. My research indicates that ketones are the key to this energy source. Since 2001, there has been at least 23 research studies done on ketones. The following is a summary of this research about ketones and the bodily need for the alternative energy source.

Ketones were first noticed in the urine of diabetic patients in the mid 19th century. They originally thought they were abnormal and undesirable by byproducts of incomplete fat oxidation. Early in the 20th century ketones became recognized as normal circulating metabolites produced by the liver and used by the body. (2)

In the 1920's a hyperketogenic diet was found remarkably effective for treatment of drug resistant epilepsy in children. In 1967, circulating ketones were found to replace glucose as the brain's major fuel during prolonged fasting. Until that time, the brain was thought to be totally dependent upon glucose. Finally, growing evidence suggests that patients with Parkinson's and Alzheimer's Disease can use ketones for their energy supply. (2)

Ketones are your body's alternative energy source. When glucose reserves are exhausted, synthesis from fats produces ketones which are then delivered to the cells to be burned for energy. However, glucose is the preferred fuel and ketones are produced only as a backup. (3) For example, when fasting or eating a very low carbohydrate diet the body uses what is usually stored as fat and converts this to energy. While it has been mentioned that the use of coconut and MCT oil helps eliminate the need for carbohydrate counting this is still a concern. If any obesity is an issue this needs to be addressed.

One particular diet which supports the ketone theory is the Atkins Diet. There have been over 50 studies which support this method of weight loss. The diet supports the value of omega3 in fish and flax seed. As well, nuts benefit the diet with good fats. Coconut has been found to be another good fat due to the fact that it contains MCT. Also extra virgin olive oil is viewed as a healhy fat. (4)

Ketones are medium chained triglycerides which do not behave like the common long chained fats. With their shorter chemical structure, they are easily absorbed and rapidly metabolized in the liver.

Affected neurons can use ketones for energy and when they are made available starving brain cells perk right up. When this fuel source is supplied on a consistent basis, remarkable changes happen. Researchers increased the ketone levels of patients with Alzheimer's for three months. In a control group of participants, with one set of subjects who did not have a change and another set who increased ketone levels, it was found that the group which experienced increased ketone levels increased cognitive scores. The other group showed a significant decline in scores. (3)

Fortunately, there are efforts being made to prepare a "super ketone" known as D-B-hydroxybutyrate, which is a ketone fuel for the brain and can be taken orally. It is not just a fuel but a "super-fuel" more efficiently producing ATP energy than glucose or fatty acid. *Ketones have to be the brain's back-up fuel.* It has protected neuronal cells in tissue culture against exposure to toxins associated with Alzheimer's or Parkinson's. (5. 6)

Therapeutic effects of ketones for the brain are old news. Ketogenic diets have been used since the 1920's to effectively prevent or reduce seizures in patients with epilepsy and a handful of studies suggest that such a diet would improve other neuro-degenerative conditions.

Recommendations from the research indicate using ketone therapy for all patients with Alzheimer's, Parkinson's, dementia, Multiple Sclerosis, Lou Gehrig's disease and other neuro-degenerative disorders. There is also evidence to suggest that it may be beneficial for people with Down Syndrome, autism and diabetes. (3)

Ketosis has been essential to a starving man's survival by the process of providing a non-glucose substrate to the brain. Ketosis is explained as the elevation of D-B-hydroxybutyrate and actoacetate. The process of ketosis saves muscle from destruction for glucose synthesis. This process gives a more efficient source of energy to the brain per unit of oxygen. The process has also been shown to decrease

19

cell death in human neuronal cultures. The observation findings raise the possibility that many neurological disorders, both genetic and acquired, might benefit by the ketosis. Another beneficial outcome from ketosis includes an increase in energy. This can be important in treating drug resistant epilepsy and in injury of anoxic states. The result of ketosis to exide co-enzyme Q and to reduce nicotinamide adenine dinucleotide phosphate (NADP) may be important in decreasing free radical damage. (7)

Parkinson's Disease appears to result from an acquired defect in the mitochondria. Again, we are in an area of neuronal damage caused by a combination of free radical damage and lack of nutrients getting to that area of the brain. So this hypotheses paper written on Ketone Bodies in 2001, seems to be working toward the conclusion that Alzheimer's and other related neuro disorders can benefit from using the ketone bodies. Basically, in research it is being discussed about how to use the ketone bodies to help with disease. They are also discussing different methods for the large-scale production of the ketone's bodies. This is another step forward that they are getting closer to the ketone mystery.(7)

As recently as December 2010, researchers published their remarkable findings in the report titled "Nutrition and Alzheimer's disease: The detrimental role of a high carbohydrate diet." A ketogenic diet was determined to be therapeutic for Alzheimer's Disease patients. This would be a very high fat diet. The reason for this type of diet to be beneficial is due to bio-availability of this high level supply of fats to repair membranes. With this type of diet leading to ketone bodies in the blood serum, they add an alternative to glucose. Ketosis was found to lead to more production of acetyl-CoA, which allows neurons to achieve a greater production of glutamine and GABA. These are vital nutrients for neurotransmission. (12)

An Introduction to the Ketogenic Diet

The Ketogenic Resource by Mynchen in the U.K. explains the ketogenic diet:

The ketogenic diet is a high fat diet which appears to help some people with epilepsy, particularly children. It is not a magic cure and is just one alternative to the various anti-epileptic drugs. The ketogenic diet may offer the advantages of more benign side effects and reduced impact on the mental development of children.

"The ketogenic diet is often regarded as a difficult regime; however, with some care and a basic understanding of what the diet aims to do, it can be reduced to a readily manageable routine. The basic aim is to switch the primary fuel used by the body from carbohydrates (like bread and sugar) to fats; this is done by increasing the intake of fats and greatly reducing the intake of carbohydrates. The difficulty is that the level of carbohydrates must be very low, and the temptation of a single sweet can upset the diet for a small child.

A typical meal might include fish and green vegetables with a mayonnaise sauce followed by fresh fruit with lashings of cream, or bacon and eggs followed by coffee and yet more cream - so the diet is not as bad as you might have feared. There are several variants of the diet; in the US, a very high ratio of fats to carbohydrates is maintained, together with a low total calorie and fluid intake; in the UK it has been usual to adopt a more relaxed regime, supplemented by MCT oil (an extract from coconuts).

The reason the ketogenic diet should reduce the level of fits is not understood; indeed many aspects of the ketogenic diet are less science and rather more black magic, and there is a need for much more research into the subject." (8)

While this information refers to epilepsy, it has been found that the ketogenic diet is a large basis for treatment and potential reversal of Alzheimer's, Parkinson's and other diseases as mentioned.

The Atkins Diet is primarily based on the powers of ketosis to cause weight loss and to help maintain weight loss. There have been many testimonies from people who have followed this diet and have found that medical issues such as diabetes, high cholesterol, and other medical issues have greatly improved.

Science of the ketogenic diet is largely based on high protein, complex carbohydrates, low sugar and high fiber. Unless other health issues indicate different levels the desirable protein intakes are considered to be best at about .8 grams per pound. Ideally, about 20 to 25 percent of the daily diet should be made up of protein. Turkey, chicken, duck, fish, beef, pork, eggs, beans, whole grains, and nuts. (9)

Fiber sources are carbohydrates which you cannot digest. Recommended intake is about 20 grams per day for women and 30 for men. Sources are beans, whole fruits and vegetables, nuts, flax seeds and whole grain products such as breads and cereals. (9)

Carbohydrates are not the enemy on a ketogenic diet. It is just best to befriend the ones who are going to help you the most. Sticking with whole grains, brown rice, Bulgar wheat, whole oats is the most beneficial. Sources for fiber are similar to the sources for carbohydrates. This is a great way to load the day with healthy choices. The key is to satisfy the sweet tooth with natural food sources. (9)

Vital to the well-being of all who choose a low carbohydrate diet is to remember that low carbohydrate does not mean no carbohydrate. Depending on personal weight management, the usual amount for weight loss for adults is about 20 grams of net carbohydrates per day to start and increasing after about a week by 5 grams per week. Once the weight goal is met, the usual recommended amount is gradually increased by about 10 net carbohydrates until weight no longer fluctuates. Net carbohydrates are the amount of carbohydrate grams minus grams of fiber. (4)

Recent research has been found to support the Mediterranean-type diet to reduce cognitive decline. (10) This type of diet is similar to the ketogenic diet. The main ingredients of the Mediterranean Diet include:

- ✓ Eating abundant amounts of whole grains, fruits, and vegetables

- ✓ Enjoying moderate portions of cheese and yogurt

- ✓ Choosing healthy fats like olive oil, nuts, avocados, and canola oil

- ✓ Drinking wine in moderation, usually with meals, if okay to do so

- ✓ Consuming fish and seafood regularly

✓ Eating small amounts of red meat only few times per month

✓ Being physically active daily (11)

With the Mediterranean diet in reference to diseases covered in this book, it is advisable to consider eliminating alcohol. There is some research which indicates that a little wine might help prevent Alzheimer's but this is an issue not yet resolved. This is due to the need to keep the brain free of any chemicals which might promote an adverse effect. As well, canola oil should also be eliminated. Vitamin and mineral needs should be met by the daily diet. Be cautious with fish and seafood due to metal toxicity. Wild salmon is considered okay.

Realistically, most people are not following a perfect diet. Supplements can be added to ensure that the proper needs for nutrition are met. This may vary by individuals and it may be helpful to consult with a health food store for more guidance. Using multiple vitamins and minerals may be another option. This all depends on individual needs.

Monitoring Ketones

In order to monitor ketosis, which is the goal in a ketogenic diets, ketone strips can be used. These are available for about $20 for 200 strips. Take one of the strips and dip in the urine. It will turn from pink to purple as soon as the body starts making a significant amount of ketones. The darker the color, the more ketones.

Check urine for ketones the first thing in the morning. Before any program is started, there will not likely be any color change at all. This is indicating that the body is making very few ketones. Start taking coconut oil and check urine in the morning and afternoon. If there are no ketones showing then it is time to consider cutting more carbohydrates. Eventually the strip will change to the purple, indicating ketones.

Bear in mind that some people achieve ketosis without this ever showing on a ketone strip. Some will just show a trace amount all the time. This is usually the case when someone has less concentrated urine, become exposed to sugars without realizing, over exercising, or metabolism of some artificial sweeteners. If weight loss or toning is noticed, this is another indicator that the body is experiencing ketosis. Desired cognitive changes are the preferred indicators of ketosis.

Results from ketosis and the use of coconut oil and/or MCT normally show up in about two weeks after starting treatment. As with all medical changes it is important to check with a doctor before beginning a regimen.

Keep a journal of ketones levels and dosages of coconut oil. This will help document progress as well as provide documentation for doctor visits. In the back of this book are sheets to help with progress. These sheets can be zoomed larger and copied to personal preferences.

References:

1. Peppard, Richard and Others, Cerebral Glucose Metabolism in Parkinson's Disease With and Without Dementia, *Archives of Neurology*, 49 (12), 1262-1268

2. VanItallie, Theodore M.D. and Nufert, Thomas B.A., Ketones: Metabolism's Ugly Duckling, *Nutrition Reviews*, October 2003, 327-341

3. Whitaker, Julian M.D. Health & Healing, October 2009

4. Westman, Eric; Phinney, Stephen; Volef, Jeff, <u>New Atkins for A New You</u>, March 2010

5. Cahill, G.F. and Others, Hormone-fuel interrelationships during fasting, *The Journal of Clinical Investigation*, 1966; 45 (11), 1751-1769

6. Cahill, George Jr. and (by invitation) Veech, Richard, Ketoacids? Good Medicine? *Transactions of the American Clinical and Climatological Association*, Vol 114, 2003

7. Veech, Richard and others, Ketone bodies, potential therapeutic uses, *IUBMB Life,* April 2001, 51 (4): 241–7

8. The Ketogenic Resource, www.mynchen.demon.co.uk

9. Harvard School of Public Health, www.hsph.harvard.edu/nutritionsource

10. Tangney, C. and others, Adherence to a Mediterranean-type dietary pattern and cognitive decline in a community population, *Am J Clin Nutr.* 2011 Mar; 93(3):601-7. Epub Dec 22, 2010

11. Oldways Mediterranean Foods Alliance (MFA) http://mediterraneanmark.org

12. Seneff S, et al, Nutrition and Alzheimer's disease: The detrimental role of a high carbohydrate diet, Eur J Intern Med (2011), doi:10.1016/j.ejim.2010.12.017

Other Conditions Which May Be Helped by Ketogenic Diets

ALS or Lou Gehrig's Disease

Lou Gehrig's Disease or Amyotrophic lateral sclerosis (ALS) attacks the motor neurons of the brain and spinal cord which control the muscles. This progressive condition affects strength, speech, swallowing and breathing, but does not affect sexual, bowel or bladder functions.

Glucose is so important to the brain function and lack of glucose causes neurons to be impaired and lose their function. With ALS the brain and spinal cord could be accessed by the use of MCT. This would not necessarily be the same portion of the brain affected by Alzheimer's. (4) This is why sometimes diseases of the brain are referred to as "diabetes of the brain" because like regular diabetes and its function with glucose, the brain can also have a similar problem.

Autism

Still a mystery to many researchers, the spectrum of autism disorders is thought to be biological with some degree of genetic origin. On one end of the spectrum we have classic autism, symptoms of which include poor language development, the inability to recognize another person's state of mind, unusual preoccupations, and repetitive behaviors. At the other end we have Asperger's Syndrome (AS), with symptoms including moderate to high intelligence in one or more areas but lack of social skills such as reading non-verbal behavior. In between are several similar disorders such as Rett Syndrome. Disorders across this spectrum affect some 1.5 million persons in the U.S., according to the Autism Society of America. (5)

Some believe that autism is caused by the failure to prune sufficient nerve cells in the two months before birth, or they may not prune correctly. Humans reach greatest brain density in the second trimester, with significant pruning of unnecessary cells in the time remaining before birth. Francesca D'Amato of Italy's National Research Center, believes that attachment disorders such as autism may be at least partially attributable to defects in the opioid or pleasure center of the brain. D'Amato hypothesizes that deficient opioid systems deny the newborn any pleasurable association with mother contact, which leads to indifference. (5)

Uta Frith of University College London has determined that autism is attributable primarily to connectivity problems rather than specific locational deficiencies. In other words, different parts of the brain simply do not work with one another. This discovery should lead to breakthroughs in treatment.(5)

Regarding the use of MCT oil for autism Arturo Volpe, M.D. has stocked MCT oil in his office to help patients with focus and mental clarity issues. While he does not claim that MCT oil is a cure for autism it can be "another little piece that is proving to play a helpful role. (6) Dr. Volpe has an online message board to help people share experiences and ask questions.

Other studies indicate a positive outcome for autism and Rett syndrome with a ketogenic diet. Such studies, while preliminary, offer hope for those who have these disorders and their families. The Department of Pediatrics at the University of Crete, Greece conducted a study, reported in 2003. A group of 30 participants between 4 and 10 years of age were placed on a ketogenic diet. 18 of 30 children demonstrated improvement in the Childhood Autism Rating Scale. (10) Another study for Rett syndrome patients included MCT oil. Treatment results showed that there it appears that there is a medical benefit for patients with Rett Syndrome. (11)

Diabetes

Diabetes is a chronic (lifelong) disease marked by high levels of blood sugar. Insulin is a hormone produced by the pancreas to control blood sugar. There are different types of diabetes. They have marked differences in monitoring and treatment.

Type 1 diabetes is the result of the body's immune system attacking insulin-producing beta cells in the pancreas. Once beta cells have been destroyed, the body make little to no insulin. This is the hormone needed for transforming glucose into energy. What ends up happening is that the blood sugar rises too high and could cause ketoacidosis. This could be life threatening. Eventually retinopathy (eye complications, including blindness), neuropathy (nerve damage) or heart disease could result. While no cure is known for diabetes there are treatments designed to help maintain blood sugar levels. In order to keep blood sugar levels healthy it may require multiple insulin injections, following a recommended diet and getting regular exercise. (7)

Type 1 diabetes is typically called "juvenile diabetes" because it usually is diagnoses in childhood or before adulthood. This does not mean that a diabetic cannot be diagnosed in adulthood. About 5 to 10 percent of diabetics are diagnosed as Type 1. Common symptoms are excessive thirst, frequent urination, blurred vision, extreme fatigue and hunger, and weight loss. There may be other illnesses where diabetes is diagnosed without the patient being aware of these symptoms. (7)

Type 2 diabetes is often called "adult onset" diabetes because it is usually detected in adulthood. Most patients are middle-aged and older. Alarmingly there is a greater occurrence of diagnoses of new cases in which the patients are adolescents and young adults. This type of diabetes is narked by insulin resistance and insulin deficiency. Insulin resistance is the body's resistance to insulin produced by the body. Insulin resistance occurs when the body makes enough insulin but not enough to get past insulin resistance. Glucose levels rise when insulin cannot transport glucose to the body's cells for energy. The same as with Type 1 diabetes retinopathy, neuropathy, and heart disease could result. (7)

Type 2 diabetes can be arrested. Complications could be prevented or delayed thanks to treatment focused on controlling blood glucose levels with a healthy diet, regular exercise, oral medications which may or may not include insulin. There is a greater chance for cardiovascular disease. Blood pressure and cholesterol checks and treatment as needed are vital. These can increase the chances of preventing heart attacks or strokes. (7)

Overweight, obesity, family history along with symptoms of excessive thirst, blurred vision, fatigue and recurring skin and urinary tract infections are indicators of a possible Type 2 diabetes patient. 90 to 95 percent of cases are Type 2 diabetics. There are an estimated 23.6 million people with diabetes and about 20 percent who have not been diagnosed. (7)

Gestational diabetes is diabetes that occurs in about 4 percent of pregnancies. The cause is unknown but common belief is that hormones for a baby's development reduce the availability to the mother's body. Insulin resistance occurs. The mother's blood sugar may rise too high. Possibly the baby could end up with a heavy birth weight and a future risk for Type 2 diabetes. The mother could get preeclampsia, requiring a Cesarean section. Treatment includes eating properly, regular exercise, testing blood sugar and possible insulin injections. (7)

Once the baby is born, gestational diabetes normally goes away. One pregnancy with this condition does not mean the next will be the same. It is possible to develop Type 1 or Type 2 diabetes while pregnant. Typical symptoms are excessive thirst, frequent urination, blurred vision, exhaustion, excessive hunger and weight loss. There may not be any symptoms. This is a case for good prenatal care. Family history of diabetes, having gestational diabetes before and overweight before pregnancy are risk factors. (7)

Focusing on diet as an important part of treatment for diabetes there are a variety of options.

Duke University conducted a study in which participants were put on a ketogenic diet and the results were remarkable. Duke researchers concluded that "lifestyle modification using low carbohydrate interventions is effective for improving and reversing type 2 diabetes." (8) Much like the ketogenic diet discussed in this book, this diet is in sync with treatment for other diseases. With notable research continuing to support the use of this method along with medications to address accessing ketones there will be more options to increase chances of recovery. While there are no definite cures this warrants further focus on such options.

Epilepsy

Mostly known for the seizures produced, epilepsy is combined effects from both mental and physical functions. Another name is seizure disorder. If there are two or more unprovoked seizures, usually epilepsy is the reason. There is a strong, yet short sure of electrical activity affecting the brain. Signs of seizures can range from jerking movements to convulsions and loss of consciousness. (12)

When medications do not seem to work for epilepsy a closely monitored ketogenic diet may be recommended. This has been going on since the 1920's. As more medications have been successful, less dietary changes have been made. It is not known why a ketogenic diet works for some and not others to prevent seizures. It is highly recommended to have a medical professional closely monitor an epilepsy patient who takes part in a ketogenic diet. (12)

Huntington's Disease

Genetic by nature, Huntington's disease (HD) is known by degeneration of brain neurons. Characterized by uncontrolled movements, loss of mental faculties and emotional upset are the result of the degeneration. Treatment of HD has been accomplished with various medications. In 2008 the drug tetrabenazine was approved for treating of writhing movements. This is the first drug approved for treatment in the U.S. With side effects of fatigue, restlessness or hyper-excitability this makes physical fitness very important. (13)

With genetic studies still at a distance there is a possible form of treatment to help HD patients. Just as with Alzheimer's and other diseases helped by a ketogenic diet, there is the same hope possible for HD. This may not work for all patients but is something to consider when looking at current options. (14)

Multiple Sclerosis

Multiple Sclerosis (MS) is the second-most common neural disease among young adults. The first is head injury. MS occurs when the immune system mistakenly identifies brain and spinal cord tissues, and particularly the myelin sheath that covers axons, as foreign invaders and attempts to get rid of them. Major symptoms can include weakness, paralysis, tingling, numbness, disturbed vision, balance and coordination problems, slurred speech, loss of bladder and bowel control, chronic pain and severe fatigue.

MS often results in disability from fatigue. Patients report an overwhelming sense of tiredness, lack of energy or a feeling of exhaustion during or after motor or mental activity. A study was made measuring regional cerebral glucose metabolism (the cerebraletabolic fluoeodeoxyglucose (CMRGlu) using PET and a tracer called F-fluorodeoxyglucose (FDG). This test determines cerebral energy metabolism related to cerebral blood flow and local synaptic activity. CMRGlu was significantly lower in MS groups. Apparently, this is another case where the glucose is not providing enough energy to the brain and body. When you feed the neurons with the triglycerides then the bodily function can be on its way to restoration of the energy level. (2)

Harvard's Rohit Bakshi shows that the brain's gray matter destruction, or neuronal death, appear to have iron deposits. This may be to blame just like the iron deposits seen with Alzheimer's Disease and Parkinson's Disease. Studies suggest that the elderly (those over 65) should avoid iron supplements. (3)

A study of the ketogenic diet in relation to ALS indicated that such a diet may "slow motor deterioration and protect motor neurons through a promoting energy production in the mitochondria of SOD1-G93A ALS mice." This effect might suggest that there is potential help for ALS with a ketogenic diet.

References:

1. Howard, P.J., PhD, The Manual for the Brain, 419-421
2. Cahill, George F. Jr. and (by invitation) Veech, Richard L., Ketoacids? Good Medicine?, Transactions of the American Clinical and Climatological Association, Vol. 114, 2003
3. Howard, P.J., PhD, The Owner's Manual for the Brain, 419-421
4. Cahill, George F. Jr. and (by invitation) Veech, Richard L.. Ketoacids? Good Medicine?, *Transactions of the American Clinical and Climatological Association*, Vol. 114, 2003
5. PET Program, 1997 by American Academy of Neurology, 1556
6. Newport, Mary M.D., *What if there was a cure for Alzheimer's Disease and no one knew?* Case Study, July 22, 2008
7. Pierce, J. Howard, PhD. *The Owner's Manual for the Brain*, 16.2, 408, 2006
8. Volpe, Arturo M.D., Coconut oil, Alzheimer's Disease, Seizures, Autism and more, November 15, 2010 http://doctorvolpe.com
9. American Diabetes Association, 1701 North Beauregard St., Alexandria, VA 22311 www.diabetes.org
10. Diabetes Health, 365 Bel Marin Keys Blvd, Suite 100, Novato, CA 94949 www.diabeteshealth.com
11. Zhao, Zhong and others, A ketogenic diet as a potential novel therapeutic intervention in amyotrophic lateral sclerosis, *BMC Neuro.*, 7:29 2006
12. Vlachonikolis, Evangeliou A. and others, Application of a ketogenic diet in children with autistic behavior: pilot study, *J Child Neurol.* Feb: 18, 2003
13. Hass, Richard H. and others, Therapeutic effects of a ketogenic diet in rett syndrome, Am J Med Genet Suppl., 1:225-46, 1986
14. Epilepsy Foundation, 8301 Professional Place, Landover MD 20785 www.epilepsyfoundation.org
15. NIH Neurological Institute, P.O. Box 5801, Bethesda, MD 20824 www.ninds.nih.gov
16. Masino, S.A. and others, Adenosine, Ketogenic Diet and Epilepsy: The Emerging Therapeutic Relationship Between Metabolism and Brain Activity, *Current Neuropharmacology,* Volume 7, Number 3, pp. 257-268(12), September 2009

Coconut Oil? Really?

Let's take a walk down coconut lane. Coconuts are seeds, versus nuts and are coined the "seed of life." With over 1,000 uses of the coconut there is no doubt that this is a much valued seed. Every part of the coconut has a purpose. From the use of the shells for non-edible purposes to the full benefits of coconut water, milk, and meat. Coconut oil is extracted from the meat of a coconut. (1) Eating the meat of the coconut is the most basic, natural way to benefit from MCT. To ensure that the best, most concentrated and exact amount of MCT coconut oil is typically used.

Using coconut oil for the benefits of MCT has been practiced for many years. In the Philippines coconut oil is called the "drugstore in a bottle." It is considered the safe oil because it does not contribute to heart disease. As a natural antioxidant, coconut oil is one of the best defenses against free radicals. This helps to prevent heart disease and clogged arteries. (1)

Referencing the studies of Dr. Mary Newport, adding about 7 teaspoons of coconut oil per meal in the daily diet has been found to work for others. If this is not the preferred route, MCT oil could be used with about 4 teaspoons once to twice daily. More MCT or coconut oil can be used. These are suggestions to be adjusted according to the individual. If side effects, such as severe diarrhea, occur then adjust the dosage to individual needs. Dr. Newport has suggested adding fish oil capsules twice daily and two servings of salmon per week. This adds to what has been found with the Ketsyn option. (2)(3) Health wise, the addition of all these components to the daily diet indicate no harm. If there are certain allergies, of course, this is an exception.

Bruce Fife, N.D. recommends a maintenance dose of 3 to 4 tablespoons per day for adults. He has taken up to 14 tablespoons a day with no problem. The main issue with this is that there may be intestinal distress and possible runny stools. He has found that there are many people who have used high amounts when they have had some serious health problems which are helped with this dosage. It is not advisable to take coconut oil all at once. Giving the body a steady dosage is always best and has found to be more beneficial. Inclusion in the daily diet is the preferred route. (1)

Dr. Newport offers the following pointers:

- MCT oil can be combined with coconut oil with the formula of 16 ounces of MCT oil to 16 ounces of coconut oil. (Found at the last update of February 2011.
- A 2" by 2" square of raw coconut could be eaten to provide about 15 grams of oil.
- Use coconut oil to saute or stir fry.
- Bake with coconut, such as macaroons, and add flaked coconut to food dishes. (2)

Other points to consider are:

- Use organic, extra-virgin coconut oil available in health food stores and from the internet.
- Avoid canola and other refined oils, which may make matters worse. Safely use olive oil but not at high heat.
- Start coconut oil gradually in the diet. Suggested is to use as much coconut oil as one would use margarine and add two more teaspoons.
- Gradually increase coconut oil until about 4 to 5 tablespoons are consumed over the course of a day.
- Use coconut oil in place of other fats and oils in recipes.

Oral use of coconut and coconut oil is one way to help with staying healthy, as well as reap benefits for Alzheimer's treatment. Topical use is also beneficial for various skin conditions. A closer look about the various treatments are found in Bruce Fife's book: <u>Coconut Cures</u>. (1)

When looking at ways to make coconut a part of the daily diet it is nice to keep things interesting. Recipes are abundant. Just keep in mind that if there are concerns over weight gain then a low carbohydrate diet is generally the option many people take. Enjoyment is still possible with restrictions. The key is keeping whole foods in the diet instead of refined, over processed foods.

Recipe resources readily found online, at the library or in book stores:

- Coconut Lover's Cookbook by Bruce Fife, N.D. Has superb reviews and every recipe with sugar has an alternative for low sugar diets.

- Grains, Greens, and Grated Coconuts by Ammini Ramachandran

- Naturally Nutritious by Nicole Kurland.

- www.cooks.com

- http://www.ecoviva.com/html/coconut-oil-recipes.html

- http://www.freecoconutrecipes.com from the Tropical Traditions resource at http://www.tropicaltraditions.com

- lowcarbfriends.com Specific coconut oil recipes are on the blog: http://www.lowcarbfriends.com/bbs/recipe-forum-sticky-threads/334903-coconut-oil-recipes-ideas.html

One of the many people I have spoken to about the use of coconut oil for Alzheimer's Disease has stayed on my mind. A woman shared that her husband had Alzheimer's Disease. She was very understandably concerned. I shared with her the values of the use of coconut oil and supplements in addition to the medications prescribed by her husbands doctor. She decided to consult the doctor and go with the conventional methods of treatment. This has been perplexing to me as the thought came to mind: *"What does she have to lose?"* Just the possibility of hope for help with this challenging disease merits a reasonable trial.

References:

1. Fife, Bruce N.D., <u>Coconut Cures, Preventing and Treating Common Health Problems with Coconut</u>, 2005

2. Newport, Mary M.D.. Coconut Oil & Alzheimer's Disease, Ketones as Fuel for Neurons. November 2009

3. Newport, Mary, M.D., *What if there was a cure for Alzheimer's Disease and no one knew?* Case study by Dr. Mary Newport, July 22, 2008

Dr. Mary Newport Puts Theory to A Test

Dr. Mary Newport conducted a case study as reported on July 22, 2008. (1) Coming from an extensive neonatology background she has experience with ketones and infants.

Dr. Newport's husband, Steve Newport, was 58 at the time of the case study report. He holds a BSBA in accounting and had been working as a bookkeeper for his wife's medical practice. As a work at home professional and parent, Steve found it more and more challenging to complete tasks with his business and home responsibilities. He eventually could not perform accounting tasks accurately. Depression, confusion, disorganization and frustration took over what was once his cheerful disposition along with well-organized and creative functioning.

Steve Newport had been diagnosed with progressive dementia in 2003. In 2004 he completed a Mild Mental Status Exam (MMSE) and was found to score in the mild range of dementia. Treatment began in 2005 with a common medication for dementia known as Aricept. A second medication, Namenda, was added a year later. In 2007 Exelon was exchanged for Aricept. An MRI report in May 2008 disclosed that Steve had what laymen refer to as "shrunken areas of the brain." This is a clear indicator of Alzheimer's Disease. With progression of the disease this brought about steadfast determination for Dr. Newport to find a way to help her husband.

Dr. Newport researched multiple journals and patents. She had found that the study on ketone bodies and their effect on dementia and other diseases hold great promise. Putting studies to the test Dr. Newport began her husband on a treatment program and joined him in this effort. Studies indicated that medium chain triglycerides (MCT) were found to produce ketones which provide energy to the brain. A ketogenic diet is typically a low carbohydrate diet. What happens is that the brain uses ketones instead of sugar for energy. This happens when people fast, are weight training, attempting to lose weight, and in certain medical treatments.

With Alzheimer's the brain is not using the neurons properly when they cannot be accessed. Insulin resistance, common to Alzheimer's, is the culprit. With a ketogenic diet the body uses the MCT oil as the source for energy. It has been found that this opens up the blood flow to the brain, increasing brain functioning at remarkable levels.

MCT oil comes from coconut or palm kernel oil. When taken in recommended dosages these oils are metabolized not as fat but for energy. This discounts the reports that coconut oil is not healthy. The main difference is that pure, non-hydrogenated and non-trans fat oil must be used. Dosage was calculated to be about 2 tablespoons of pure virgin coconut oil per each meal. It can be eaten straight or mixed into food.

Results from a 60 day report indicated that Steve was able to go from not being able to draw a picture of the face of a clock to drawing one by the 37th day. He has come along nicely. Possibly he would have to have occupational therapy but overall has shown remarkable improvement. Something which also may have helped was eating salmon twice weekly and taking fish oil supplements.

Others have reported marked improvement with the use of MCT oil and continued research is expected to prove promising. Dr. Newport has appealed for assistance on her blog for research funding for the studies of Dr. Richard Veech and others. She states the urgent need for finding for Alzheimer's, Parkinson's, Huntington's Chorea, Multiple Schlerosis, ALS, Diabetes, and other conditions which are characterized by a defect in glucose transport. (3)

Since this study Dr. Newport has gone on to report progress of her husband, her case subject. In her website: coconutketones.com and in her blog coconutketones.blogspot.com Dr. Newport opens up opportunities for others to share their experiences with the use of coconut oil for Alzheimer's treatment.

Update As of February 2011

Dr. Newport posted an update on her husband's progress in February of 2011. After over 32 months of improvement by Steve Newport there are both ups and downs. The improvements outweigh the downside. Steve has held on to prior improvements and quality of life has greatly increased. (2)

MRI reporting as of April 2010 indicates that Steve has been considered stable as compared to the marked atrophy previously reported in 2008. This means success has been found with treatments. As of February 2011: Steve's gait has continued to be normal. He continues to run and also does fast walking with his wife. He no longer has visual problems related to reading. This actually stopped within four months of starting on MCT and coconut oils. He now reads occasionally and is able to pronounce even complex words. (2)

Mild tremors may occur if Steve is late for his oils. Nothing has changed with this response. Steve did have a depression after his father's death in spring 2010 but he has improved over time. He is able to use the riding lawn mower, vaccuum, and helps with shredding records for the duration of an hour or longer, showing an improvement with becoming less distracted. (2)

Steve is now able to keep up a conversation with others. Family members have noticed a steady improvement. In September 2009 Steve would often wear one shoe or sock. The new report is that he now wears shoes and socks in pairs. Steve is able to recall out of county trips and major events. (2)

After volunteering for about a year at the hospital where Dr. Newport works, Steve wanted a paying job. He started working with a social program for dementia patients. While he is a client he volunteers his time to do some shredding and vacuuming. He has not obtained paid employment. Steve still has his winning personality and unique sense of humor. (2)

There have been some setbacks which seem to be related to medications due to illnesses. These setbacks have been a disorientation to person and place in the evening. He has had some concern when he sees images in the dark windows at night. He started having some confusion about persons and places. Possible responses to having been sick with a viral infection and taking prednisone for gout may go along with his difficulties at night. He has had considerable improvement since he is no longer on the medicines. (2)

Dr. Newport reported that all is not perfect. She believes Steve would not score in the 18-20 range on the MMSE. As a participant in the Eli Lilly gamma secretase trial Steve suffered side effects and may not have been on the trial medication for long. While he had the MMSE scores to qualify for this study the outcome was that he received a drug to make matters worse. (2)

Dr. Newport reports that the current dosage of oils is an equal mixture of MCT and coconut oil, administered at three tablespoons per meal. 15 ml fish oil is given daily. This is a mixture of 5 ml cod liver oil and 10 ml fish oil. (2)

It has taken several months for Steve to be able to gain tolerance to MCT and coconut oil. It is important to take these dosages in order for the brain to benefit. Dr. Newport reported that the fish oil helps with a vital part of Alzheimer's treatment. Alzheimer's patients are generally low in DHA (one of the elongated

38

omega-3's). There may be a deficiency in a liver enzyme in the way vegetable sourced omega-3 fatty acids are processed. It becomes vital to have a marine source of omega-3 fatty acids. While coconut oil has some omaga-6 fatty acids it does not contain amega-3. (2)

With regard to mixing MCT and coconut oils Dr. Newport conveys that while they started with replacing fats with coconut oil, including cooking, Steve consumed about 2 tablespoons for each breakfast and dinner meal. An increase to about 4 teaspoons of MCT oil was added to breakfast and dinner. Steve's ketone levels peaked about three hours after breakfast. By dinner the ketones were barely present. Levels rose after dinner and continued to rise at three hours. MCT oil caused the levels to peak in 90 minutes and be non-existant in three hours. This made it necessary to consume coconut oil at each meal.

Dr. Veech's guidance in July 2008 was to add MCT oil for higher levels. The coconut oil is still used to keep ketones present longer. The other factor is the antimicrobial benefits of coconut oil. Dr. Newport mentions research about a virus which may be a cause for Alzheimer's. This is a herpes simplex virus which may affect people of the ApoE4+ genotype. Lauric acid, which is in coconut oil, kills the herpes family of viruses. Diarrhea occurred with increase of MCT oil. When taken with food this is less likely to happen. The mixture of four parts MCT and three parts coconut oil was changed to 50:50.

It isn't easy to mix the MCT and coconut oils together without some pointers from Dr. Newport. If MCT and coconut oil are mixed they will stay in liquid form. They are kept this way at room temperature. Placing the container of coconut oil in a bucket of hot water for about twenty minutes will cause the oil to melt. You may have to change the water to keep it hot.

Mixing equal portions of each oil in a quart jar will serve to keep a good supply on hand. Be sure to shake before each use. She also suggests adding 1-2 teaspoons liquid soy or egg lecithin to act as an emusifier for each full jar. Lecithin is also good for the brain. Gradually use the mixture at a starting level of 1 teaspoon for 2-3 times per day.

Dietary Considerations

As important as the oils used in the daily diet there is also consideration to be given to the rest of the diet followed by the Newport family. Their diet mainly consists of whole, unprocessed foods and low carbohydrates. Fish is eaten several times a week, poultry, some beef, fresh or fresh frozen fruits and vegetables. Whole grain bread, rice and pasta are eaten in small amounts. Eggs, while dairy, goat milk and goat cheese, coconut oil and coconut milk are all important. Avoiding lunch meats which have artificial colors and preservatives and eating organic, free range poultry is most helpful. While there may be a treat now and then the need to follow a healthy eating regimen is important. Steve takes Exelon and Namenda prescriptions and certain supplements. he takes them are various times so he is not taking too many pills at once. Powder forms can be blended with liquid yogurt at breakfast. He takes:

- ✓ B vitamins: Folic acid, folate, niacin, B12, pantethine (B5) powder
- ✓ Oil based forms of vitamin E (400 IU mixed tocopherols) and vitamin D3 (2500 IU per day)
- ✓ Vitamin C (2000 mg per day)
- ✓ Niacinamide (3000 mg per day)
- ✓ Turmeric
- ✓ Magnesium
- ✓ Acetyl-L carnitine
- ✓ CoQ10 as ubiquinol
- ✓ D-ribose powder
- ✓ Phosphatidyl serine
- ✓ Chromium
- ✓ Zinc
- ✓ L-lysine powder about 3 grams per day and valacyclovir 1 gram per day to try to suppress outbreaks of fever blisters.
- ✓ Caffeine 400 mg per day

Dr. Newport reported that since the time the news was reported about Steve in October 2008 the word has spread. It has reached over 700,000 people via the website www.coconutketones.com and continuous publication of her original article and summaries.

Numerous caregivers have reported directly to Dr. Newport and/or various message boards about others who have known the remarkable improvements such as Steve has experienced. While they are not all about cognitive test scores they are about trials and tribulations. Even if there is not an improvement shown they are encouraged to keep up with the oils and journaling. When people stop using the oils they may come to realize that there was more improvement than noticed. (2)

She has heard from people in regard to other forms of dementia and how there have been marked improvements. Dr. Newport stated: "We are very thankful that

Steve is among those who have improved and wish with all of our hearts that this would be the case for everyone." (2)

The wife of a man diagnosed with dementia after a heart operation was left to the choice of a nursing home and refused to go that route. She took him home and after learning from Dr. Newport about her husband, she decided to start her husband on the same form of treatment. Within three hours her husband started responding after just one treatment. Today he is able to get on the computer and continue in his ministry. (5,6,7)

Dr. Newport offers the latest regarding other research about ketone ester. She states that there are deveopements with Dr. Veech's research. In 2009 human toxiciology testing was completed. This followed with FDA approval for use of the ketone ester for healthy adults. In 2011 there is a study of "rowers and couch potatoes" in Oxford England. This is using the ketone ester to check the effects on cognitive and physical performance. This is again, for otherwise healthy people. (2)

Funding is still greatly needed in order to produce ester for clinical trials of Alzheimer's patients. It is with great hope that a financial contributor will come forward. This could be by charity, government, pharmaceutical company, or for private company. Ideally, it will be best to keep the costs down, making this affordable for everybody who needs it. With the creation of the ketone ester there will be a significant difference in ketone therapies without the use of MCT or coconut oil. (2)

A new website due out in late 2011 cognatenutritionals.com will be provided for those interested in the results of Dr. Theodore VanItallie research. He is working on a liquid nutrition supplement. This will provide a measured dose of coconut and MCT oil. (2)

Watch for the Book: *Alzheimer's: What If There Was a Cure? The Story of Ketones*, by Mary T. Newport, M.D., anticipated publication date in August 2011, Basic Health Publications, Inc. (3)

References:

1. Newport, Mary M.D. *What if there was a cure for Alzheimer's Disease and no one knew?* Case study, July 22, 2008. All references therein the case study report.

2. Newport, Mary M.D. Steve Newport-Coconut Oil Case Study, Update February 2011

3. Newport, Mary M.D. Blog: coconutketones.blogspot.com

4. Flett, Bruce YouTube video on the page of GrandmaCarolFlett

5. Flett, Carol, Blog: *Can God Use Facebook to Answer Prayers?* www.everydaychristian.com/blogs/post/9322/

6. Flett, Carol and Bruce, www.godleadsusalong.com/

7. Flett, Carol http://healthimpactnews.com/

Plan for Action and Success

We have discussed theories, discoveries and tests to get to this point. Let is take a look at how it all comes together. There are some tools which may be helpful as you venture into a trial of an Alzheimer's prevention or treatment program. The first thing to do is to make a doctors appointment. Work a plan with the doctor.

Setting up the tool box, you will need:

➤ **Digital or Video Recorder**

➤ **Charts for keeping track of dosages**

➤ **Journal (can be done on the computer)**

➤ **Pharmaceutical grade, non hydrogenated, no trans fat virgin coconut oil**

➤ **MCT oil**

➤ **Vitamins and Minerals**

➤ **Ketone Testing Strips**

➤ **Acidophilus Capsules**

➤ **Fish Oil Capsules**

➤ **Healthy Foods as mentioned**

At the beginning of the process, record the person who is undergoing treatment. Interview them, if possible. Make notes in the journal as to dates and progress. This will help to provide great documentation for not only progress but also research. As the patient undergoes changes be sure to video document these milestones. Record the way the person walks and talks. Document facial expressions and physical changes.

When starting out with the coconut and MCT oil regimen, start slow. Too high of a dosage at the beginning may result in loose bowels. This can be very painful and urgent. Starting out with small doses, about one third of the desired dosage, lets the body get used to changes. Eventually the goal is to take about 4-6 tablespoons of coconut oil per day. This is best to spread over the course of the day. Dr. Newport suggests mixing equal parts of coconut oil and MCT oil. (2)(3)

Coconut oil can be used in place of cooking oils, butter, shortenings. It can be baked or cooked or eaten as is. Since it will smoke at temperatures exceed 350 degrees it is best to add some olive or peanut oil when cooking. For baking in foods coconut oil can be used at higher temperatures. You can put coconut oil in hot cereal, salad dressings, and just about anything to satisfy personal tastes. Not only the oil but also coconut flakes, milk, ice cream, macaroons and even fresh coconut chunks can be enjoyed.(2)

Incorporating coconut oil with recipes is easy to accomplish. The nice flavor goes will with other cooking products. Just be cautious about overeating, especially since coconut oil regimens can cause weight gain. This can be counteracted with dietary controls such as sticking with whole foods. Add two fish oil capsules to the daily diet. The Omega-3 benefits as well as adding other Omega-3 rich foods can help put that edge out there for success.

Acidophilus may be helpful, especially if there is a tendency toward irritable bowel issues. Lactobacillus acidophilus is an active ingredient in some, but not all yogurt. This lactic acid producing bacteria helps aid digestion. Health food stores usually have acidophilus supplements in capsule, liquid and powder form. Normally it is best to take this supplement before meals or at least an hour after meals.(1)

Some people may also want to add a fiber supplement. If so, be sure to use this in conjunction with meals. Do not take fiber supplements at the same time of day as medications. Some people take fiber supplements at bedtime. Be certain to drink plenty of water to encourage bulking and prevent choking.

Check ketones using the ketone strips. These are available at pharmacies and are often behind the counter. They do not require a prescription. Once the body is making a significant amount of ketones, the strips will turn purple. The best time to check is first thing in the morning. This can be done daily, even more than once per day. If the strips do not show a color change after about two weeks, it may be a sign of eating too many carbohydrates. Dietary changes may need to take place. Be sure to work with the doctor regarding ketone treatment.

Check online message boards mutual support of others in their ongoing trials and tribulations. Keeping that connection is very helpful as it is easy to feel alone. There are so many people searching for answers and this is a great way to link. Check out local resources via hospitals and community groups. Not everybody is online and this can help add that human aspect which is often needed for encouragement.

References:

1. Health Central, 2300 Wilson Blvd., #600, Arlington, VA 22201
   www.healthcentral.com

2. Newport, Mary T. M.D., Coconut Oil Dietary Guidelines and Suggestions, September 2009 coconutketones.com

3. Newport, Mary M.D., Steve Newport-Coconut Oil Case Study, Update February 2011

Dear Caregiver,

At the end of this book, you will find charts to help keep track of the ketone levels and dosages of MCT and coconut oils. You will also have pages to use for journaling. I have also added resource information for places to turn for alternative health information.

Please send us a letter explaining how the program developed for your family member. Let us know how everything turned out. Tell of any new results we many not know about. We would like to know as you are documenting the coconut oil treatment about how they are tolerating the regime.

Let us know how they are coping with the process. We care very much about other people struggling to regain their health. We would like to know how you are doing. Having lived the past 50 years with failing health and discovering much success with this MCT oil and coconut oil, I am very much interested how other folks cope and I would love to hear your success stories. Learning how others have finally found better health is a future I wish for all of you. You can mail this letter to us at:

Allen Golden
Seek Health Ltd
2008 West Broadway
Suite 152
Council Bluffs, IA 51501

allenkgolden@yahoo.com

Good Luck Patients, Caregivers, and God Bless You All!

Sincerely,

Allen K. Golden

Alternative Health Resources

The Alliance for Natural Health USA
1350 Connecticut Ave NW, 5th Floor
Washington, DC 20036
Phone: (800)230-2762
www.anh-usa.org

American Association of Naturopathic Physicians
Phone: (866)538-2267
www.naturopathic.org

American College for Advancement in Medicine, ACAM
Phone: (888)439-6891
www.acam.org

American Academy of Environmental Medicine, AAEM
Phone: (316)684-5500
www.aaem.com

Coconut Oil and Ketones
Blog of Mary Newport, M.D.
http://coconutketones.blogspot.com

Cornerstone Therapy Center
Dr. Murphy
8031 West Center Rd
Suite 321
Omaha, NE 68124
(402)392-1766

Dr. McCleary-Renowned Doctor and Author
www.drmccleary.com

Green Acres Natural Foods Market
805 South Main St.
Council Bluffs, IA 51503
(712)323-5799
www.greenacresnaturalfoods.com

How Healthy Eating Can Change Your Life - "Let Food Be Your Medicine"
www.healthy-eating-politics.com

International College Integrative Medicine
Phone: (866)464-5226
www.icimed.com

Meridian Valley Laboratory
Phone: (425)271-8689
www.meridianvalleylab.com

Nutrition & Healing online
www.WrightNewsletter.com

Dr. Richard Schultze
https://www.herbdoc.com
Tahoma Clinic for Appointments Only
Phone: (425)264-0059

Tahoma Clinic Dispensary
to order supplements and products only
Phone: (888)893-6878
www.tahomadispensary.com

Whitaker Wellness Institute
http://www.whitakerwellness.com

Other Alzheimer's Resources

Alzheimer's Foundation of America
322 8th Ave., 7th Fl.
New York, NY 10001
Phone: (866)AFA-8484
www.alzfdn.org

The Alzheimer Spouse
www.thealzheimerspouse.com

Alzheimer's Books and Materials
The Alzheimer's Store
3197 Trout Place Road
Cumming, GA 30041
Phone: (800) 752.3238
http://shop.alzstore.com/storefront.aspx

Best Alzheimer's Products provides references to anything from art therapy
information to caregiver information, research abstracts and more.
www.best-alzheimers-products.com/research.html

Elder Care Resources
Phone (800)677-1116
www.eldercare.gov

Family Caregiver Alliance
180 Montgomery St, Ste 900
San Francisco, CA 94104
Phone: (800)445-8106
www.caregiver.org

Help Guide for Alzheimer's Patients and Caregivers
http://www.helpguide.org/

Low Carber Forum
http://forum.lowcarber.org **in connection with** www.lowcarb.ca

National Alliance for Caregiving
4720 Montgomery Lane, 2nd Floor
Bethesda, MD 20814
www.caregiving.org

National Family Caregiver's Association
www.thefamilycaregiver.org

The Weston A. Price Foundation
PMB Box 106-380 4200 Wisconsin Avenue, NW
Washington, DC 20016
www.westonaprice.org

Pointers for Cooking:

⋏ Melt coconut oil and mix with equal parts MCT oil for easier blending.

⋏ Do not deep fry fish as this destroys omega3's.

⋏ Use coconut oil when a recipe calls for another fat.

⋏ Coconut oil smokes at higher temperatures. Keep at about 300 degrees and add equal portions of olive oil. Then the temperature can be raised to 350 for stove top cooking.

⋏ Mix coconut oil with any store-bought salad dressing. This lends a nice flavor, which does not overpower the taste.

⋏ Flax seed meal, hazelnut meal, and almond meal can be used in place of flour in standard recipes. You may need to adjust to taste.

⋏ Soy flour may be used sparingly. Too much soy may upset the system.

⋏ Experiment with various recipes to find where coconut oil can be added. You might be surprised at how this ingredient blends right in with foods.

⋏ Kefir is a liquid drink with yogurt and can be used in smoothies or for doses of coconut oil and MCT oil.

⋏ Coconut milk is now readily available in grocery stores and can be used in place of regular milk.

⋏ Sprinkle coconut flakes on anything from fruit to fish. Unsweetened coconut flakes are available in whole food stores.

⋏ Do not use whole flax seeds as the real nutritional benefits come through in the meal. They must be ground. You can use a coffee grinder or buy flax seed meal.

⋏ The internet is full of recipes for coconut products. Refer to the list of sites mentioned in the coconut oil section of this book.

Simply quick recipes:

Smoothie

2 1/2 cups plain yogurt
1 cup frozen strawberries or other sweet fruit
1 banana
Stevia to equal 1 tablespoon, or other sweetening agent to taste
2 tablespoons melted coconut oil or add MCT/coconut oil combination
Can add any other fruits as desired

Starting with liquids and sweeteners blend until smooth. Add remaining ingredients and blend until mixed well. May add crushed ice if desired.

Simply Quick Anytime Snack

1/4 cup flax meal
1/2 teaspoon baking powder
Sweetener to equal 2 teaspoons
1 teaspoon cinnamon
1 large egg
1 tablespoon solid or liquid coconut oil

Mix all ingredients in a microwave safe, 8 ounce or higher, bowl

Place in microwave and start at one minute. If somewhat doughy then continue for 15 second increments until desired consistency. Can be toasted.

Variations:

Add dash of garlic powder in place of cinnamon and omit sweetener to use for buns.

Experiment with other flavorings. I like to use unsweetened coconut flakes and to serve with raspberry jam.

Can be made into pancakes by adding milk to batter consistency and cooking on griddle.

Can be cooked in oven at 325 for about 15 minutes.

Caregiver Stress Management

Caregivers and Alzheimer's patients alike are vulnerable to stress. Stress affects health and personal relationships. If your resources to handle situations are low or depleted, there is more vulnerability to become ill or to have much confusion.

Ideally, one of the best ways to manage stress is to build an arsenal of awareness which is stocked daily. Some of the items needed in the arsenal are:

- ◆ Assertiveness. By practicing the art of saying "no" when asked to do something which throws off your balance of energy and availability.

- ◆ Feelings Checks. By communicating each day about how you feel. This clears the air and helps you recognize the value of your feelings. If feelings are numb then this is a sign of too much stress.

- ◆ Have fun! Life is too short to spend each day without enjoyment. Take the time to play games, read, go to movies, go out to eat and do whatever you truly enjoy.

- ◆ Exercise. This does not mean you have to run a marathon. Go outside for fresh air ad take a walk in the neighborhood or go to a mall or gym. Senior center tend to have discount programs and many options to make exercise fun.

- ◆ Journal. Keep a journal for yourself along with encouraging the family to do the same. This provides release, insight, problem solving, and personal documentation.

- ◆ Flexibility. Sometimes it seems like a day is full of compromises. When caring for others you often have to change plans to meet their needs. Accepting that each day has surprising moments makes it easier to handle whatever comes your way.

- ◆ Nutritional meals. Feeding your internal arsenal helps to build stamina and energy stores. Treat yourself to foods you like and make meals a featured event.

◆ **Medication and Supplements.** If there are medications which you must be on, be sure to take them consistently. Supplement the diet with necessary vitamins and minerals.

◆ **Engagement.** Involving your family member who has Alzheimer's in activities you enjoy will make their lives better. This helps to build strong, healthy relationships. Getting others involved with activities helps for socialization.

◆ **Respite.** Take time away from your family, if possible. Respite care can be provided by other family members or friends. If this is not possible then check into respite care programs in the community. Adult day care may be an option, as an example.

◆ **Reality Checking.** There are bound to be some days which are frustrating. Accepting that there are going to be these days will help you let the stress slide. Be good to yourself. If it is a stinky day then just do your best to roll with the flow.

Making a game out of feelings identification makes keeping in touch with reality fun. This can be a family event and can be incorporated into charades, as one example. Take care of yourselves and recognize that you are the most valuable resource to your loved ones. Make it fun to discover and get in touch with feelings. On the next page is a list of feelings words to help you get started.

<u>Resources</u>

There are some wonderful feelings charts and games on the following websites:

toolsforeducators.com

freeprintablebehaviorcharts.com

These are the most common feelings to use for the feelings game:

Afraid

Angry

Annoyed

Anxious

Bored

Cheerful

Confused

Curious

Embarrassed

Excited

Frightened

Grumpy

Guilty

Jealous

Joyful

Happy

Lonely

Loving

Nervous

Proud

Sad

Scared

Shy

Sick

Silly

Surprised

Tired

Worried

Bibliography

Alzheimer's Association, 225 N. Michigan Ave., Fl. 17, Chicago, IL 60601-7633
www.alz.org

American Diabetes Association, 1701 North Beauregard St., Alexandria, VA 22311
www.diabetes.org

American Health Assistance Foundation, 22512 Gateway Center Drive,
Clarksburg, MD 20871 www.ahaf.org

Cahill, George F. Jr. and (by invitation) Veech, Richard L.. Ketoacids? Good
Medicine?, *Transactions of the American Clinical and Climatological Association,*
Vol. 114, 2003

Cahill, G.F. and Others, Hormone-fuel interrelationships during fasting, *The
Journal of Clinical Investigation,* 1966; 45 (11), 1751-1769

Centers for Disease Control and Prevention, 1600 Clifton Rd., Atlanta, GA 30333
www.cdc.gov

de la Monte, SM and Wands, JR, Alzheimer's disease is type 3 diabetes-evidence
reviewed. *J Diabetes Sci Technol.* 2008 Nov;2(6):1101-13

Diabetes Health, 365 Bel Marin Keys Blvd, Suite 100, Novato, CA 94949
www.diabeteshealth.com

Dunnet, Stephen B. and others, Cell therapy in Parkinson's disease – stop or go?
Nature Reviews-Neuroscience, 365-369

Epilepsy Foundation, 8301 Professional Place, Landover MD 20785
www.epilepsyfoundation.org

Fife, Bruce N.D., Coconut Cures, Preventing and Treating Common Health
Problems with Coconut, 2005

Flett, Bruce YouTube video on the page of GrandmaCarolFlett

Flett, Carol, Blog: *Can God Use Facebook to Answer Prayers?*
www.everydaychristian.com/blogs/post/9322/

Flett, Carol and Bruce, www.godleadsusalong.com/

Flett, Carol http://healthimpactnews.com/

Flett, Carol, How to treat dementia and Alzheimer's with coconut oil, *http://mental-health.helium.com*

www.freeprintablebehaviorcharts.com

Gabuzda, Dana and Other, Inhibition of Energy Metabolism Alters the Processing off Amyloid Precursor Protein and Induces a Potentially Amyloidogenicc Derivative, *The Journal of Biological Chemistry,* 1994. 13623-13628

Gerngross, T.U. National Biotechnology, 1999, 17, 541-542

Graham, D.I,. and Others, Acta Neurochirurgica, Wein, Supp. 66, 96-102

Hamosh, M. and Hamosh, P., Lipoprotein lipase: Its physiological and clinical significance. *Mol Aspects Med* 1983, 6, 199-289

Hamosh, Margit PhD and Others, Lipids in milk and first steps in their digestion, *Feeding the Normal Infant,* 2001

Harvard School of Public Health, *www.hsph.harvard.edu/nutritionsource*

Hass, Richard H. and others, Therapeutic effects of a ketogenic diet in rett syndrome, *Am J Med Genet Suppl., 1:225-46, 1986*

Health Central, 2300 Wilson Blvd., #600, Arlington, VA 22201
www.healthcentral.com

Honea, Robyn and others, Progressive regional atrophy in normal adults with a maternal history of Alzheimer disease, *Neurology*, Vol. 76 no. 9 822-829, March 1, 2011

Howard, Pierce J., PhD, <u>The Owner's Manual for the Brain</u>, 1999

Kalaria, R.N. and Others, The New York Academy of Sciences 695, 190-193
The Ketogenic Resource, www.mynchen.demon.co.uk/

Masino, S.A. and others, Adenosine, Ketogenic Diet and Epilepsy: The Emerging Therapeutic Relationship Between Metabolism and Brain Activity, *Current Neuropharmacology,* Volume 7, Number 3, pp. 257-268(12), September 2009

Marambaud, Philippe and Others, Resveratrol Promotes Clearance of Alzheimer's DiseaseAmyloidB-Peptides, *J. Biol. Chem.* Vol. 280; Issue 45: 37377-37382

Masino, S.A. and others, Adenosine, Ketogenic Diet and Epilepsy: The Emerging Therapeutic Relationship Between Metabolism and Brain Activity, *Current Neuropharmacology,* Volume 7, Number 3, pp. 257-268(12), September 2009 Monell Chemical Senses Center. "Natural Compound In Extra-virgin Olive Oil -- Oleocanthal -- May Help Prevent, Treat Alzheimer's." ScienceDaily September 29, 2009

Newport, Mary T. M.D., Coconut Oil Dietary Guidelines and Suggestions, September 2009 www.coconutketones.com

Newport, Mary M.D. Steve Newport-Coconut Oil Case Study, Update February 2011

Newport, Mary M.D. Blog: coconutketones.blogspot.com

Newport, Mary M.D.. Coconut Oil & Alzheimer's Disease, Ketones as Fuel for Neurons. November 2009

Newport, Mary, M.D., *What if there was a cure for Alzheimer's Disease and no one knew?* Case study by Dr. Mary Newport, July 22, 2008

NIH Neurological Institute, P.O. Box 5801, Bethesda, MD 20824 www.ninds.nih.gov

Oldways Mediterranean Foods Alliance (MFA) http://mediterraneanmark.org

Oz, Mehmet www.doctoroz.com

Patton, S. Keenan, T.W., The milk fat globule membrane, *Biochem Biophys Acta,* 1975, 415, 273-309

Peppard, Richard and Others, Cerebral Glucose Metabolism in Parkinson's Disease With and Without Dementia, *Archives of Neurology,* 49 (12), 1262-1268

PET Program, 1997 by American Academy of Neurology, 1556

Seneff S, et al, Nutrition and Alzheimer's disease: The detrimental role of a high carbohydrate diet, *Eur J Intern Med* (2011), doi:10.1016/j.ejim.2010.12.017

Shallenberger, Frank M.D., Real Cures Newsletter, December 2009

Tangney, C. and others, Adherence to a Mediterranean-type dietary pattern and cognitive decline in a community population, *Am J Clin Nutr.* 2011 Mar; 93(3):601-7. Epub Dec 22, 2010

www.toolsforeducators.com

VanItallie, Theodore M.D. and Nufert, Thomas B.A., Ketones: Metabolism's Ugly Duckling, *Nutrition Reviews*, October 2003, 327-341

Veech, Richard and others, Ketone bodies, potential therapeutic uses, *IUBMB Life,* April 2001, 51 (4): 241–7

Volpe, Arturo M.D., Coconut oil, Alzheimer's Disease, Seizures, Autism and more, November 15, 2010 http://doctorvolpe.com

Vlachonikolis, Evangeliou A. and others, Application of a ketogenic diet in children with autistic behavior: pilot study, *J Child Neurol.* Feb: 18, 2003
Westman, Eric; Phinney, Stephen; Volef, Jeff, New Atkins for A New You, March 2010

Whitaker, Julian M.D. Health & Healing, October 2009

Whitaker, Julian M.D. www.whitakerwellness.com

Wright, Jonathan, A three-pronged attack on Alzheimer's, *Nutrition and Healing Newletters,* September 23, 2009

Wright, Jonathan, *Nutrition & Healing Newsletters,* Vol. 16, Issue 8, October 2009

Zhao, Zhong and others, A ketogenic diet as a potential novel therapeutic intervention in amyotrophic lateral sclerosis, *BMC Neuro.*, 7:29 2006

Date/Time	Ketone Level	Coconut/MCT Dosage	Notes/Response

Date/Time	Ketone Level	Coconut/MCT Dosage	Notes/Response

Date/Time	Ketone Level	Coconut/MCT Dosage	Notes/Response

Date/Time	Ketone Level	Coconut/MCT Dosage	Notes/Response

Date/Time	Ketone Level	Coconut/MCT Dosage	Notes/Response

Date/Time	Ketone Level	Coconut/MCT Dosage	Notes/Response

Journal for recording thoughts, noting progress, feelings, and pretty much anything.

Journal for recording thoughts, noting progress, feelings, and pretty much anything.

Journal for recording thoughts, noting progress, feelings, and pretty much anything.

Journal for recording thoughts, noting progress, feelings, and pretty much anything.

Journal for recording thoughts, noting progress, feelings, and pretty much anything.

Journal for recording thoughts, noting progress, feelings, and pretty much anything.

Journal for recording thoughts, noting progress, feelings, and pretty much anything.

Journal for recording thoughts, noting progress, feelings, and pretty much anything.

Journal for recording thoughts, noting progress, feelings, and pretty much anything.

Journal for recording thoughts, noting progress, feelings, and pretty much anything.

Journal for recording thoughts, noting progress, feelings, and pretty much anything.

Journal for recording thoughts, noting progress, feelings, and pretty much anything.

Journal for recording thoughts, noting progress, feelings, and pretty much anything.

Journal for recording thoughts, noting progress, feelings, and pretty much anything.

Journal for recording thoughts, noting progress, feelings, and pretty much anything.

Journal for recording thoughts, noting progress, feelings, and pretty much anything.

Journal for recording thoughts, noting progress, feelings, and pretty much anything.

Journal for recording thoughts, noting progress, feelings, and pretty much anything.

Journal for recording thoughts, noting progress, feelings, and pretty much anything.

Journal for recording thoughts, noting progress, feelings, and pretty much anything.

Journal for recording thoughts, noting progress, feelings, and pretty much anything.

Journal for recording thoughts, noting progress, feelings, and pretty much anything.

Journal for recording thoughts, noting progress, feelings, and pretty much anything.

Journal for recording thoughts, noting progress, feelings, and pretty much anything.

Journal for recording thoughts, noting progress, feelings, and pretty much anything.

Journal for recording thoughts, noting progress, feelings, and pretty much anything.

Journal for recording thoughts, noting progress, feelings, and pretty much anything.

Journal for recording thoughts, noting progress, feelings, and pretty much anything.

Journal for recording thoughts, noting progress, feelings, and pretty much anything.

Journal for recording thoughts, noting progress, feelings, and pretty much anything.

Journal for recording thoughts, noting progress, feelings, and pretty much anything.

Journal for recording thoughts, noting progress, feelings, and pretty much anything.

Journal for recording thoughts, noting progress, feelings, and pretty much anything.

Journal for recording thoughts, noting progress, feelings, and pretty much anything.

Journal for recording thoughts, noting progress, feelings, and pretty much anything.

Journal for recording thoughts, noting progress, feelings, and pretty much anything.

Journal for recording thoughts, noting progress, feelings, and pretty much anything.

Journal for recording thoughts, noting progress, feelings, and pretty much anything.

Journal for recording thoughts, noting progress, feelings, and pretty much anything.

Journal for recording thoughts, noting progress, feelings, and pretty much anything.

Date	Medications	Vitamins and Minerals

Date	Medications	Vitamins and Minerals

About the Author:

Allen Golden is a man who has experience with healthy alternatives to traditional medicine. When he learned how it is was possible to combat Alzheimer's Disease he moved forward to find out more. Spending countless hours doing medical research, Golden was able to find significant journal articles and other information to shed light on his research.

Knowing that it is now possible to treat Alzheimer's and many other diseases with some very simple ingredients, along with pharmaceuticals, he had to share the wealth of his findings. Once the fire was in his heart he simply had to find more information to support this theory.

It is his sincere hope that people who are battling Alzheimer's and other diseases will be able to try alternatives and find success. While there are no absolute guarantees, these findings foster hope in the never-ending battle with Alzheimer's Disease.